Ketogenic Diet
Make Ahead Freezer Meals & Snacks

Don't Be A Slave To Your Diet

Meals At Your Fingertips
Ready When YOU Are!

By Skye Howard RD LD

Published December 2014 - SCG Publishing
This Edition February 2016

ISBN-13: 978-1530132782

ISBN-10: 1530132789

DISCLAIMER

Disclaimer and Terms of Use: Every effort has been made to ensure that the information in this book is accurate and complete, however, the author and the publisher do not warrant the accuracy of the information and text contained within the book due to the rapidly changing nature of science, research, known and unknown facts and internet. The Author and the publisher do not hold any responsibility for errors, omissions or contrary interpretation of the subject matter herein. This book is presented solely for motivational and informational purposes only. Consult your doctor before going on any diet or exercise plan.

CONTENTS

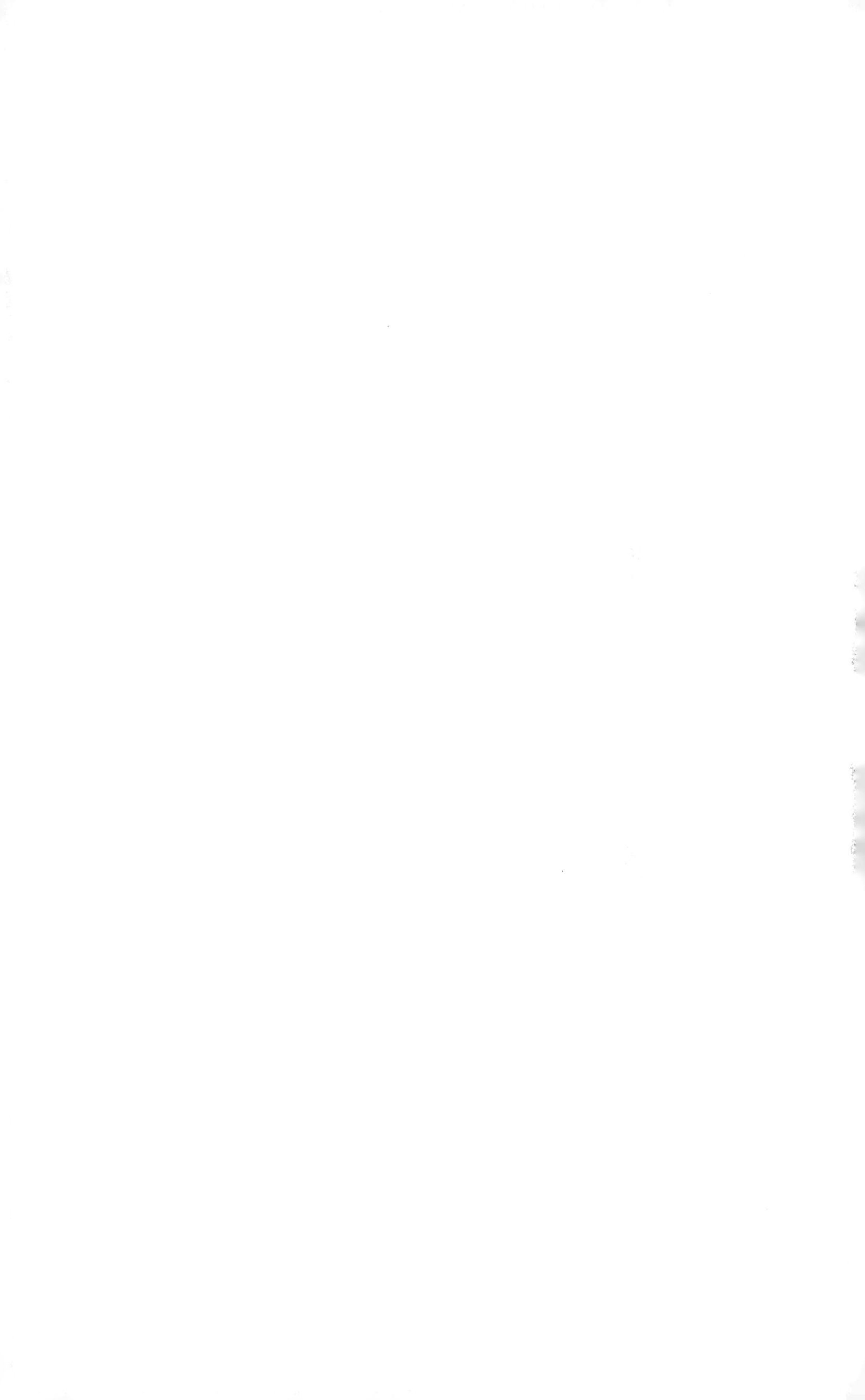

INTRODUCTION

The Ketogenic Diet can be demanding as it takes a lot of meal preparation and counting of nutritional values. Those who are not used to spending a lot of time in the kitchen will find it challenging.

The Keto Diet Make Ahead Freezer Meals & Snacks is perfect for those with limited free time, allowing for bulk meal preparation and then very little work to do when meals are needed.

This recipe book includes 45 true Ketogenic recipes that can be made in advance to cater to those with busy lifestyles. Although this diet can be challenging due its strictness in carbohydrate intake, these recipes have been developed from a registered and licensed dietician that are easy to prepare and full of flavor.

Features of this Dietician-Approved Ketogenic Cookbook include:

- 45 recipes developed and approved by a dietician that are full of flavor and color that follow the Ketogenic diet
- Simple freezer meal and use instructions for every recipe
- Recipe suggestions that are unique and personalized
- Nutrient analysis for every recipe, including total calories, total fat, total net carbohydrates and total protein
- Nine recipe categories
- Homemade, unique recipes such as Crustless Pizza, Chicken Avocado Casserole and Bacon Cheeseburger Pie
- Inclusion of avocado, a nutrition powerhouse for the brain
- Inclusion of Stevia, a natural sweetener and healthy baking ingredients, such as ground almond and coconut flour.

HOW THE KETOGENIC DIET WORKS

The Ketogenic diet is composed of high fat, adequate protein and low carbohydrates, approximately 20 grams per day on average

The body converts carbohydrates into glucose for energy. By keeping the level of carbohydrates very low, the body is forced to burn fats for its energy source instead. This is done by the liver, which converts fatty acids into ketones, which becomes the new energy source. When the level of ketone bodies in the blood becomes elevated, the body is then in a state of ketosis.

The state of ketosis takes approximately 3 days to achieve. Side effects, known as "Keto Flu", will be felt in the first few days as the body adjusts to the new diet. This is usually proof that the body is in ketosis, but to ensure that ketosis has been reached, ketostix can be purchased from a pharmacy to check if ketones are being excreted in urine. Once they are, the body is in ketosis. Care should then be taken against dehydration by drinking a lot of water and adding salt to food.

To be successful on the Keto Diet, hunger should be avoided. This is easy on a diet full of delicious food full of flavor and fats, but be aware to eat regularly to avoid carbohydrate cravings.

To receive personalized individual nutritional advice on the Ketogenic Diet and the proper ratio of fat, carbohydrates and protein, please consult with your local Registered Dietician. For medical advice, please consult your healthcare physician.

SOUPS

COCONUT CURRY PEANUT SOUP

Makes: 4 servings

All you need:

3/4 cup creamy peanut butter
2 cups low-sodium chicken broth
2 tbsp. curry paste, Madras
1 can (13 2/3 oz) light Coconut milk, unsweetened
1 can (14 ½ oz) fire-roasted diced tomatoes
2 cups shredded rotisserie chicken, skin removed

All you do:

Whisk broth and curry paste until smooth.
Heat in a saucepan over medium-high heat until boiling.
Slowly whisk in coconut milk and peanut butter, and simmer for 2 to 3 minutes.
Stir in canned tomatoes with liquid and chicken.
Add salt, to taste.

Freezing Instructions:

Let soup cool at room temperature.
Pour into plastic food storage container and label and date.
Store in the freezer for 2-3 months.

To serve:

Remove from freezer and let thaw in refrigerator overnight.

Heat through then add chopped roasted peanuts and garnish with lime wedges, if desired.

Nutritional Information (Per serving):

Calories: 527
Total fat: 37 g
Total carbohydrate: 10 g
Protein: 35 g

CHEESY RUEBEN SOUP

Makes: 14 servings
Serving size: 1 cup

All you need:

2 cloves garlic, minced
1 medium onion, diced
3 tbsp butter
2 celery ribs, diced
1 lb corned beef, chopped
1 cup sauerkraut
4 cups beef stock
1 tsp caraway seeds
1 tsp sea salt
¾ tsp black pepper
1½ cups Swiss cheese, grated
2 cups heavy cream

All you do:

Sauté chopped onions, garlic, celery and butter over medium-high heat until caramelized.
Transfer to a crockpot on high heat.
Add sauerkraut, beef stock, corned beef, and seasonings to crock-pot.
Cook, covered, on high for 4 hours, or on low for 6-8 hours.
Add Swiss cheese and cream and cook for another hour.

Freezing Instructions:

Let soup cool at room temperature.
Pour into plastic food storage container and label and date.
Store in the freezer for 2-3 months.

To serve:

Remove from freezer and let thaw in refrigerator overnight. Heat through and enjoy!

Nutritional Information (Per serving):

Calories: 225
Fat: 18.5 g
Carbohydrates: 4 net g
Protein: 11.5 g

BROCCOLI CHEDDAR SOUP

Makes: 10 servings

All you need:

2 tsp salt
3 cups chicken broth, low sodium
½ large yellow onion, chopped
2 small broccoli heads, cut into florets
1 avocado
1 cup cheddar cheese, shredded
3 cups heavy whipping cream

All you do:

Combine broth, salt, chopped onion and broccoli in a large saucepan and heat until simmering.
Cover pan and continue to simmer until broccoli is crisp-tender, about 10 minutes.
Place cooked ingredients and avocado into a food processor and pulse until desired consistency.
Return the same saucepan to stovetop over medium heat.
Add in the dairy ingredients and bring to a low simmer for 5 minutes, stirring frequently.

Freezing Instructions:

Let soup cool at room temperature.
Pour into plastic food storage container and label and date.
Store in the freezer for 2-3 months.

To serve:

Remove from freezer and let thaw in refrigerator overnight.
Heat through and enjoy!

Nutritional Information (Per serving):

Calories: 326
Fat: 32 g
Carbohydrates: 3 g
Protein: 5 g

CHEESY CAULIFLOWER BACON SOUP

Makes: 6 servings

All you need:

1 cauliflower head
2 tbsp olive oil
1 medium onion
4 slices bacon
12 oz. Cheddar cheese
1 tsp ground thyme
3 cups chicken broth
¼ cup heavy cream
1 oz Parmesan cheese
1 tbsp minced garlic

All you do:

Chop cauliflower into small florets and place on a baking sheet rubbed with oil.
Season the cauliflower with salt and pepper and bake at 375 degrees for 30 minutes or until cauliflower is golden brown.
While cauliflower is baking, pan-fry or microwave the bacon until crisp.
Save the bacon drippings and pan-fry the chopped onion in the grease.
Sprinkle in the dried thyme and cook until all the flavors come together, for almost 1 minute.
Pour in the broth then transfer the roasted cauliflower to the saucepan next.
Bring to a low boil for approximately 15 minutes.
Pour ingredients into a food processor or blender, or use an immersion stick blender.
Once a soup consistency is formed, gently stir in the cheese until melted followed by the crispy chopped bacon and heavy cream.

Freezing Instructions:

Let soup cool at room temperature.
Pour into plastic food storage container and label and date.
Store in the freezer for 2-3 months.

To serve:

Remove from freezer and let thaw in refrigerator overnight.
Heat through and enjoy!

Nutritional Information (Per serving):

Calories: 337
Fat: 25 g
Carbohydrates: 11 g
Protein: 18 g

CHICKEN

BAKED SPICY CHICKEN

Makes: 2 servings

ll you need:

2 boneless, skinless, chicken breasts, 4 oz each
4 oz cheddar cheese
2 oz jalapeno slices (optional)
Pinch of salt and half pinch of pepper
4 slices bacon

All you do:

Season thawed chicken with salt and pepper, as desired.
Sprinkle with cheese, 2 oz per chicken breast.
Add jalapeno slices, if desired.
Cut the bacon in half and drape over the chicken.

Freezing Instructions:

Transfer to a foil-lined pan and cover with foil.
Label and date foil with cooking instructions.
Place in freezer for up to 6 months.

To serve:

Remove from freezer and let thaw in refrigerator overnight.
Bake at 350°F for 30-45 minutes or until done.
Place under broil for approximately two minutes for crisper bacon, if desired.

Nutritional Information (Per serving):

Calories: 296
Fat: 16.5 grams
Carbohydrates: <1 gram
Protein: 35 grams

SIMPLE FREEZER CHICKEN

Makes: 8 servings
Serving size: 1 cup

All you need:

32 oz boneless, skinless chicken breasts
Salt and pepper, to taste
Clean knife
Raw meat cutting board
Canola oil spray

All you do:

Slice the chicken into pieces approximately 1-inch in thickness size.
Spray a 9x13 baking dish with oil spray; assemble chicken breasts in pan.
Add a pinch of salt and ½ pinch of pepper and distribute over all the chicken breasts.
Note: Consider wearing gloves for prevention of cross contamination.
Bake chicken at 350°F for approximately 30 minutes.

Freezing instructions:

Transfer to a bowl, cover with plastic wrap and allow to cool completely in the refrigerator.
Use gallon size zip top bags to store the chicken and lay flat on a freezer shelf.
Once chicken is frozen, shake the zip top bag to break up chicken and squeeze any excess air from bag then reseal.

To use:

Simply take out of freezer and let thaw in refrigerator before use.

Nutritional Information (Per serving):

Calories: 125
Fat: 1.5 g
Carbohydrates: 0 g
Protein: 26 g

PRE-COOKED CHICKEN RECIPES

Makes: 8 servings

All you need:

32 oz boneless, skinless chicken, cooked

All you do:

Add chicken to food processor and pulse until crumbled or shredded.
Use in chicken salad or for chicken nuggets

Freezing Instructions:

Add pulsed chicken into freezer ziploc bags and remove any excess air.
Label and date the bags and store in freezer for up to 6 months.

To use:

Once needed, remove from freezer and let thaw in refrigerator overnight.

Nutritional Information (Per serving):

Calories: 125
Fat: 1.5 g
Carbohydrates: 0 g
Protein: 26 g

AVOCADO CHICKEN BAKE

Makes: 8 servings

All you need:

8 boneless chicken thighs, cooked
4 small avocados, cut, pitted, sliced
1 medium onion, chopped or finely diced
1 medium pepper, sliced
8 oz sour cream, regular
8 oz cheddar cheese
1 tbsp Frank's Red Hot Sauce (chile pepper sauce)
Salt and pepper, to taste

All you do:

Preheat oven to 350°F.
Bake chicken thighs for 1 hour or until juices run clear.
Prepare avocados according to instructions below.
Grease a baking dish and add avocado slices to the bottom. Save any extra for later.
Pan-fry the pre-sliced pepper and onions over medium-high heat until caramelized.
Shred chicken with a fork.
Add the remaining ingredients to the shredded chicken, including the extra avocado and pour over the bottom layer of avocado slices.
Bake for 20 minutes.

Freezing Instructions:

Once casserole is cooled, cover dish tightly with cling wrap then foil.
Label and date the dish then store safely in freezer for up to 6 months.

To serve:

Let thaw overnight in refrigerator then heat through in oven.

How to Open an Avocado:

Place the avocado lengthwise on a secure surface.
Hold the avocado securely with one hand.
Use a sharp knife to cut lengthwise around the avocado.
Let the knife follow the contour of the avocado by pressing the knife blade into the flesh touching the large pit.
Twist the two avocado halves by pulling the lengthwise pieces apart gently to avoid bruising.
Use the knife to remove the pit from the avocado then whack the knife firmly into the pit. Slowly but firmly twist the knife and the pit will be easily removed from the avocado half
Make slits lengthwise into the avocado flesh.
Scoop out the avocado slices with a spoon.

Nutritional Information (Per serving):

Calories: 549
Fat: 40 g
Carbohydrate: 13 g
Fiber: 7 g
Protein: 39 g

MONTEREY CHICKEN CASSEROLE

Makes: 8 servings

All you need:

8 boneless, skinless, chicken breasts
1 cup sour cream
4 oz green chiles, diced
4 tsp taco seasoning mix
16 oz green salsa

To serve:

8 oz Monterey jack cheese
4 stalks green onions, diced

All you do:

Slice chicken breasts into even chunks.
Cook the chicken breast chunks in a pan at 350°F for approximately 30 minutes.
Pour cooked chicken into a bowl and toss together with taco seasoning.
Pour taco chicken into a casserole dish.
Mix sour cream, chilies and salsa together and pour over chicken.

Freezing Instructions:

Let casserole cool completely, and then cover with cling wrap then foil wrap.
Place in freezer.

To serve:

Let thaw in refrigerator overnight.
Cook for 25 minutes at 350°F.
Shred the Monterey Jack cheese while the chicken is cooking.
Once the chicken is done, remove and cover in cheese and cook for 5 minutes longer.
Let cool, cut into pieces, transfer to plastic food storage containers and garnish with green onions.

Nutritional Information (Per serving):

Calories: 351
Fat: 17 grams
Carbohydrate: 7 grams
Fiber: 1 gram
Protein: 34 grams

COCONUT THAI CROCK POT CHICKEN

Makes: 12 servings

All you need:

3 cans of coconut milk
3 tbsp sriracha (hot Thai chile sauce)
6 tbsp pesto
½ cup cilantro
3 tbsp soy sauce
3 x 4 oz boneless, skinless chicken breasts cut into strips
12 x 4oz boneless chicken thighs cut in halves
3 ziploc bags
4 tbsp fish sauce

All you do:

First, add a can of coconut milk to each ziploc bag.
Add the next four ingredients evenly per bag. (Note: Do not add fish sauce until cooking).
Seal bag and shake until mixed well.
Add chicken pieces evenly per bag.

Freezing Instructions:

Remove any remaining air and seal bag.
Label the bag, date and cooking instructions below.
Place bag in the freezer until needed.

To serve:

Add the frozen meal into crockpot or stovetop.
Cook on high in crock-pot for 4-6 hours or on medium-high heat over stovetop.
Occasionally stir over stovetop.

After cooked through, stir in fish sauce and let cook for another 15 minutes.
Add salt to taste (optional).
Serve over a bed of steamed non-starchy vegetables.

Nutritional Information (Per serving):

Calories: 388
Fat: 27.5 g
Carbohydrates: 4 g
Protein: 26.5 g

CHICKEN AND BROCCOLI BAKE

Makes: 6 servings.

All you need:

1½ lbs boneless, skinless, chicken breast (4 oz each)
1 tsp salt
8 oz cream cheese
1 cup chicken broth
¼ cup heavy cream
1 tsp mustard powder, ground
1 lb broccoli florets, chopped
1 cup cheddar cheese, shredded

All you do:

Season chicken breasts with a pinch or two of salt then bake for approximately 30 minutes at 350°F.
While the chicken cooks, add chopped broccoli to a steamer and cook until crisp-tender.
Heat the cream and broth together over medium-high heat in a medium saucepan.
Whisk in cream cheese until smooth then stir in mustard; set aside.
Let chicken cool for a few minutes then chop into small even pieces, about 1-inch thickness.
Add the chicken, broccoli, creamy cheese and ½ cup of cheddar cheese to the liquid mix.
Pour into a casserole dish (that has a lid if available) and sprinkle the remaining cheese on top.
Bake until cheese starts to bubble, approximately 20 minutes.

Freezing Instructions:

After chicken has cooled, cover tightly with foil then label and date recipe. Cover with lid and store in freezer.

To serve:

Let chicken thaw overnight in refrigerator and then heat through in oven before serving.

Nutritional Information (Per serving):

Calories: 346
Fat: 22 g
Carbohydrates: 3.2 g
Protein: 7.5 g

BEEF

CHUCK ROAST ONION AND MUSHROOMS

Makes: 8 servings

All you need:

2 lbs beef chuck arm roast, 1/8" fat, cut into 1¾ inch pieces
1 can regular cream of mushroom soup
1 pkg. onion soup mix
1 can Diet Sprite
Add any non-starchy veggies, as desired (carrots, cauliflower, onions, and peppers are good choices)

All you do:

Add meat to casserole dish.
In a separate bowl, stir together cream of mushroom soup and onion soup mix.
Pour mixture over meat.
Add 1 can Diet Sprite to the dish.

Freezing Instructions:

Cover tightly and place in freezer.

To serve:
Take out of freezer and let thaw in refrigerator overnight.
Place all contents into crock-pot.
Cook on low for 8-10 hours or on high for at least 4 hours.
Turn off and let side on warm for 30 minutes before serving, to allow all juices to set into meat.

Nutritional Information (Per serving):

Calories: 400
Fat: 25 g
Carbohydrates: 6 g
Protein: 35 g

GOAT CHEESE SPINACH LOAF

Makes: 6 servings
Serving size: Approximately 5 oz

All you need:

2 lbs ground beef, 70/30% fat
2 large eggs
3 cloves minced garlic
3 green onions, chopped
1 large yellow onion, diced
Large handful of fresh spinach
4 oz crumbled goat cheese
2 tbsp tomato paste

Seasonings:

All you need:

Pinch of cayenne pepper, optional
1-2 tsp oregano
1 tsp salt
½ tsp pepper
1 rosemary sprig

All you do:

Preheat oven to 425°F.
Using hands, mix together eggs and meat well.
Add in green onions, garlic and other onions; mix well with a wooden spoon or hands.
Lay plastic wrap flat on countertop and add meat on top.
Flatten meatloaf and shape into a rectangle.

Spread fresh spinach and crumbled cheese in the middle of the meatloaf.
Fold meat over like a pastry pinwheel into a meat roll.
Place in a baking dish and spread tomato paste all over the top.
Add rosemary sprig on top.
Bake for approx. 30-45 minutes.
Cook for approximately one hour.
Note: Omit tomato paste to lower total carbohydrates.

Freezing Instructions:

Let cool at room temperature.
Cut into 6 slices and a delicious cheesy spinach mixture will appear.
Add slices into individually wrapped or a large freezer Ziploc bag.
Label and date and store in the freezer for up to 6 months.

To serve:

Remove from freezer and let thaw in refrigerator for at least 8 hours or overnight.
Heat through in the oven.

Nutritional Information (Per serving):

Calories: 520
Fat: 34 g
Carbohydrates: 4.7 g
Protein: 45.6 g

FREEZE IN A FLASH MEATBALLS

Makes: 13 servings
Serving size: 3 meatballs

All you need:

2 lb ground beef, 70/30 fat%
2 lb ground pork, 80/20 fat%
1 medium yellow onion, grated
8 cloves garlic, minced
½ cup fresh parsley, roughly chopped
4 tsp dried oregano
4 tsp sea salt
2 tsp black pepper

All you do:

Preheat oven to 350°F.
Use hands to combine meat in a large bowl in addition to the remaining ingredients.
Once mixed well, form your meatballs.
Place onto a sprayed or baking sheet lined with parchment paper.
Note: You will need two baking sheets as the recipe makes approximately 40 meatballs.
Bake for 17-20 minutes.

Freezing Instructions:

Once meatballs are cooled, add meatballs in a single layer to a freezer Ziploc bag for faster freezing.
Label the bag and freeze for up to 3 months.

To serve:

To prepare, let thaw in refrigerator overnight.
Add your sauce of choice, such as marinara or pesto to the meatballs and heat through.

Nutritional Information (Per serving):

Calories: 379
Fat: 27 g
Carbohydrates: 1.7 g
Protein: 30 g

BACON CHEESEBURGER PIE

Makes: 6 servings

All you need:

1 lb. ground beef, 80/20 fat%
1 large yellow onion, diced
6 slices thick-cut bacon, bite-sized
3 large eggs
½ cup mayo or full fat plain yogurt
½ cup half-and-half
2 cups 2%-milk fat cheddar cheese, shredded
1 tsp garlic powder
½ tsp pepper

All you do:

Preheat oven to 350°F.
Pan-fry cut bacon until crispy. Remove from heat and cool.
Discard all bacon drippings except 2 tsp from the pan.
Add ground beef, diced onion and garlic powder to pan and cook until beef is no longer pink.
While beef is browning, mix together eggs, half-and-half and mayo or yogurt. Add in cheese and a pinch of pepper to the mayo mixture.
Strain the ground beef fat drippings and then add the bacon back into the pan and mix.
Press the ground beef mixture into a pie dish.
Pour egg mixture over it and bake for approximately 45 minutes.

Freezing Instructions:

Allow pie dish to cool then wrap tightly with cling wrap then foil. Place in freezer and store safely for up to 6 months.

To serve:

Remove from freezer and let thaw in refrigerator overnight. Heat through in oven then enjoy!

Serving Suggestion:

Serve with spaghetti squash instead of pasta for a low-carb meal.

Nutritional Information (Per serving):

Calories: 501
Fat: 39 g
Carbohydrates: 1.8 g
Protein: 32 g

CHEESEBURGER AND CONDIMENTS SALAD

Makes: 6 servings
Serving size: 4 oz

All you need:

6 x 4 oz hamburger patties, precooked (thawed), 70/30% fat
Toppings:

- Lettuce
- Tomato
- Onion
- Bacon crumbles
- Jalapenos
- Avocados
- Mayonnaise

All you do:

Break up precooked hamburgers with your hands.
In an individual serving bowl, add hamburger pieces and desired add-ons. Stir up all ingredients and add mayo or mustard to the bowl for added creaminess.

Nutritional Information (Per serving, meat only):

Calories: 305
Fat: 20.2 g
Carbohydrates: 0 g
Protein: 29 g

BEEF STROGANOFF

Makes: 4 servings

All you need:

2 tbsp butter
1 lb. beef chuck, 2-inch cubes
2 tbsp green onions, finely chopped

To serve:

1 cup mixed mushrooms, sliced
1 tsp Dijon mustard
½ can beef broth, lower sodium
¼ cup white wine
2 tbsp regular sour cream
Guar gum: optional to thicken beef broth

All you do:

Heat butter in pan, brown beef and onions and let cool at room temperature.

Freezing Instructions:

Place the cooked beef into a freezer ziploc bag.
Label and date the bag with cooking instructions.
Place in freezer and store safely up to 6 months.

To serve:

Remove from freezer and let thaw in refrigerator overnight.
Pour beef and onion mixture into pan over medium-high heat. Set beef aside.
Stir guar gum (if desired) into pan juices, add beef broth and bring to simmering.
Add mustard, mushrooms, sour cream and white wine.
Cover the pan and continue to simmer for 30 more minutes or until thickened.

Nutritional Information (Per serving):

Calories: 215
Fat: 11 g
Carbohydrates: 4 g
Protein: 25 g

PORK

PORK TACO SALAD

Makes: 6 servings
Serving size: 5 oz

All you need:

32 oz ground pork
6 tsp taco seasoning mix
Pinch of cayenne pepper, to taste

For serving:

9 oz cheddar cheese, shredded
6 oz regular sour cream
6 oz salsa
6 Romaine or green lettuce leaves

All you do:

Brown the pork over medium-high heat on stovetop.
Stir in taco seasoning and cayenne pepper.

Freezing Instructions:

Allow pork to cool at room temperature.
Add pork into 6 separate containers.
Place the containers in freezer.

To serve:

To thaw, place container (s) in refrigerator overnight.
Heat through over the stovetop or microwave.
Top with cheddar cheese and let melt.
Serve with desired condiments.

Nutritional Information (Per serving):

Calories: 647
Fat: 51 g
Carbohydrate: 5 g
Protein: 38 g

CROCK POT PAPRIKA PORK TENDERLOIN

Makes: 6 servings
Serving size: 5 oz

All you need:

1½ lb pork tenderloin
1 cup chicken stock
½ cup mild salsa
2 tbsp paprika
1 tbsp oregano
1-2 pinches of salt
Pinch of pepper, optional

All you do:

Stir all ingredients together and pour over pork in a slow cooker.
Cook on high for 4 hours or on low for 8-10 hours.
Use a fork to shred the pork then let sit until all juices are absorbed.

Freezing Instructions:

Once meat cools to room temperature, add pork into freezer ziploc plastic bags.
Release any excess air and lay flat in freezer.
Label and date before storing in the freezer.

To serve:

Remove bag from freezer and let thaw in refrigerator overnight.
Put contents into saucepan and heat on low-medium heat, to avoid overcooking.

Nutritional Information (Per serving):

Calories: 160
Fat: 8.2 g
Carbohydrates: 2.4 g
Protein: 21.7g

CIDER PORK CHOPS

Makes: 15 servings
Serving size: 3.2 oz

All you need:

18 pork chops
4 tbsp soy sauce
½ cup apple cider vinegar
½ cup Stevia
½ tsp pepper
½ tsp ginger

All you do:

Preheat oven to 350°F.
Add all of the ingredients other than the pork chops to a food processor and process.
Place the pork chops in a greased pan and pour the marinade mixture over it.
Cook for 30 minutes in oven, then flip over and cook for 30 additional minutes.
Remove pork chops and let cool.

Freezing Instructions:

Chop the pork chops into desired serving size and divide into ziploc freezer bags.
Lay flat and remove any excess air.
Label and date the bags and lay flat in the freezer.

To serve:

Let thaw overnight in refrigerator.
Heat through as desired.

Serving Suggestion:

Since pork chops are lean, pair them with a side higher in fat.
Add extra cheese or sour cream to increase fat content.

Nutritional Information (Approximately 3.2 oz):

Calories: 326
Fat: 25 g
Carbohydrates: 0 g
Protein: 23 g

BOSTON PORK CARNITAS

Makes: 16 servings
Serving size: 5 oz

All you need:

8 lbs Boston pork butt
2 tbsp bacon grease (use butter if necessary)
1 large onion
2 tbsp cumin
2 tbsp thyme
2 tbsp chili powder
1 tbsp salt
1 tbsp pepper
4 tbsp minced garlic
1 cup water or chicken stock

All you do:

Spread bacon grease in crockpot.
Line the bottom of the crockpot with sliced onion and minced garlic.
Remove any unwanted fat from the pork and make a crisscross pattern on the fatty layer.
Using hands, evenly rub spices all over the meat.
Add 1 cup water or chicken stock to crock-pot.
Cook on low for 8-10 hours to result in tender meat.

Freezing Instructions:

Let meat cool completely. Place in pre-labeled freezer bags, remove excess air and lay flat in freezer.

To serve:

Take out freezer bag (s) and let thaw in refrigerator.
Heat through on stovetop or microwave.
Add toppings as desired, including cheese, sour cream, lettuce, avocado and salsa.

Nutritional Information (Per serving):

Calories: 265
Fat: 9 g
Carbohydrates: 0 g
Protein: 8 g

SEAFOOD

TUNA EGG SALAD

Makes: 7 servings
Total time: 10 min Prep: 5 min Cook: 5 min

All you need:

7 cans of tuna in water, strained
3/4 cup mayo
2/3 cup celery
1/3 cup green pepper
3 green onions, diced
3/4 cup relish, sugar-free
3 large eggs

All you do:

Hard-boil all the eggs then set aside until cooled.
Strain water from canned tuna and break it up with a fork.
Add all ingredients together and mix.

Freezing Instructions:

Store in an airtight container in the freezer for up to 1 week for best quality.

To serve:

Let thaw in the refrigerator.
Great for a work lunch.

Nutritional Information (Per serving):

Calories: 363
Fat: 27 g
Carbohydrate: 2 g
Fiber: 1 g
Protein: 29 g

ALMOND FLOUR FISH TACOS

Makes: 4 servings
Serving size: 2 tacos

All you need:

Canola oil, for frying
1 bag of pork rinds, ground
3-4 fish fillet 4 oz each (This recipe works well with tilapia, halibut or cod fillets)
2 eggs, lightly beaten

For serving:

½ cup regular mayonnaise
1 chipotle pepper, chopped
Pinch of salt and half pinch of black pepper
1-2 tbsp unsalted butter
1 small green cabbage, shredded (use only 1 cup, store remaining)
1 carrot, shredded
8 almond flour tortillas (Recipe provided under Bread Recipes p.80)
1 jalapeno, thinly sliced
¼ cup roughly chopped cilantro leaves
½ cup regular feta, crumbled
Lime wedges, for garnish

All you do:

Heat 2-3 inches of vegetable oil in a large saucepan to 350°F.
In two small bowls, add pork rinds to one and eggs to the other.
Cut fish fillets into bite-sized strips and dip into egg batter then pork rinds.

In batches, drop the fish pieces into the hot oil and fry until golden brown.
Place fried fish on a paper towel on a plate to discard any extra fat.

Freezing Instructions:

Let fish nuggets cool at room temperature.
Place nuggets into a freezer ziploc bag. Label and date the bag with cooking instructions.
Store in freezer for up to 1-2 months.

To serve:

Remove fish from freezer and let thaw overnight in the refrigerator.
Heat fish nuggets through in the oven.
In a food processor, blend mayonnaise and chipotle peppers until smooth; refrigerate.
Pan-fry cabbage and carrots in the butter on medium-high heat for 2-3 minutes.
Add a pinch of salt to the cabbage and carrots and transfer to a small bowl.
Drizzle the mayo chipotle dressing on top and the condiments, including jalapeno, onion, cilantro and queso fresco with lime juice.
Spoon some of the cabbage mixture into the center of the tortilla then top with the heated fish pieces.
Enjoy!

Note:

To lower fat and protein content, simply halve or omit the pork rinds.

To add some spice, add a dash of cayenne pepper to the pork rinds.

Nutritional Information (Per serving):

Calories: 587
Fat: 58 g
Carbohydrates: 10 g
Protein: 45 g

COCONUT RED PEPPER SHRIMP

Makes: 6 servings
Serving size: 1 cup

All you need:

1½ lbs raw shrimp, peeled, deveined
¼ cup canola oil
¼ large onion, diced
1 garlic clove, minced
¼ cup canned, roasted red pepper
14 oz. can diced tomatoes

For serving:

1 cup coconut milk, unsweetened
2 tbsp hot sauce
2 tbsp freshly squeezed, lime juice
¼ cup fresh cilantro, roughly chopped
Pinch of salt and pepper, to taste

All you need:

Sauté onions in canola oil over medium-high heat until translucent and soft.
Lower heat to and stir in garlic and peppers and cook for an additional 10 minutes.
Add diced tomatoes with liquid, deveined shrimp and fresh cilantro.
Once shrimp is opaque, remove from heat and let cool at room temperature.

Freezing Instructions:

Add shrimp mixture to casserole dish and cover tightly with cling wrap then foil.
Label and date the dish with cooking instructions and place in freezer for up to 3 months.

To serve:

Remove from freezer and let thaw in refrigerator.
Pour coconut milk and hot sauce mixture over the shrimp and heat through in the oven until hot.
Add freshly squeezed lime juice and seasonings for added flavoring.
Serve with garnished fresh cilantro, optional.

Serving suggestion:

Pair with a light beer, if desired.

Nutritional Information (Per serving):

Calories: 294
Fat: 19 g
Carbohydrates: 5 g
Protein: 24 g

CHEESY FISH NUGGETS

Makes: 5 servings
Serving size: 5 fish nuggets

All you need:

½ cup ground pork rinds
½ cup parmesan cheese, shredded
Seasonings (salt/pepper/cayenne pepper/garlic powder) to taste
1 large egg
1 tbsp heavy cream
3 Tilapia fillets, 4-oz each or other fish fillets such as cod or halibut
2-3 tbsp olive oil

All you do:

Process pork rinds until a powder forms.
Mix rind power, parmesan cheese and spices together in one bowl.
Mix wet ingredients, egg and cream, in another.
Chop the fish into 1-inch thickness pieces.
Dip fish first in egg, then in pork rind/cheese mixture to coat.
Coat a pan with the oil and heat over medium-high.
Add in coated fish and cook until both sides are golden brown.

Freezing Instructions:

Let fish nuggets cool at room temperature then add to a freezer ziploc bag.
Label and date the nuggets with cooking instructions and place in freezer for up to 3 months.

To serve:

Remove from freezer and let heat in oven until ready to serve hot.

Nutritional Information (Per serving):

Calories: 377
Fat: 25 g
Carbohydrates: 1 g
Protein: 38 g

ITALIAN

ALMOND FLOUR PIZZA CRUST

Makes: 8 slices
Serving size: 2 slices (1/4 of pizza)

All you need:

2 cup shredded mozzarella cheese (or a mix of parmesan and colby)
7 tbsp almond flour
1 large egg
1 tbsp Italian seasoning
1 tsp garlic powder or 1-2 garlic cloves, minced
Pinch of basil, optional
Any sauce desired

All you do:

In a large bowl, add cheeses and microwave until just melted.
Gradually stir in almond flour just until moistened.
Let cool; add in egg and spices.
Knead with hands until dough forms.
Form into a ball.

Freezing Instructions:

Wrap dough ball in cling wrap.
Place the pizza dough in freezer for up to 3 months.

To use:

Take dough out in the morning for an evening dinner.
Preheat oven to 450°F.
Spray a large pizza stone or pizza pan. Spread crust mixture on pizza stone or pan. Note: Mixture should hold a shape.
Add sauce and toppings. Bake until cheese is bubbly and crust is golden brown.
Take out of oven and cool for 10-15 minutes.

Nutritional Information (Per serving):

Calories: 323
Fat: 25 g
Carbohydrate: 4 g
Protein: 19 g

CHEESY COCONUT GNOCCHI

Makes: 4 servings

All you need:

3 large eggs
4 tbsp coconut flour
4 tbsp parmesan cheese, finely grated
1 tsp garlic powder, optional
¼ tsp salt
1 tbsp Italian seasoning

All you do:

In a food processor or mixing bowl, mix flour, eggs, cheese and seasoning until the dough forms.
Dough should be slightly sticky and thick.
If dough is not thick, add a little more coconut flour.
Divide dough in half and roll into 2 long sausage shapes
Wrap each sausage in cling wrap and store in refrigerator for a minimum of 30 minutes or chill overnight.

Freezing Instructions:

Wrap dough in foil and label and date.

To use:

Let thaw overnight in refrigerator.
Dice rolls into 1/2 inch pieces and roll into small balls, flattening slightly.
Bring salted water to a boil and add one sausage roll of diced gnocchi into boiling water, adding 2-3 pieces at a time to avoid sticking.

Do not stir.
Once cooked, gnocchi will rise to the top.
Gently remove with a slotted spoon and set in a bowl aside.

Serving Suggestions:

Cover with your favorite sauce. Pairs well with marinara sauce.
For added protein, serve with grilled meat or chicken.

Nutritional Information (Per serving):

Calories: 107.5
Fat: 38 g
Carbohydrates: 5 g
Protein: 8 g

SKIP THE CRUST PIZZA

Makes: 6 servings

All you need:

8 oz package of regular cream cheese, softened
2 large eggs
¼ tsp black pepper
1 tsp garlic powder
¼ cup parmesan cheese, grated

Topping when serving:

All you need:

½ cup pizza sauce
1½ cup mozzarella cheese, shredded
Optional: pepperoni, ham, sausage, mushrooms, and peppers
Pinch of garlic powder, optional

All you do:

Preheat oven to 350°F.
Lightly spray a 9x13-pan with canola spray.
In a large bowl, mix cream cheese, eggs, garlic powder and parmesan cheese until smooth.
Spread into baking pan.
Bake for approximately 12-15 minutes, or until lightly golden brown.
Allow crust to cool for 10 minutes

Freezing Instructions:

Once crust is cool, wrap pan with cling wrap then foil.
Label and date the recipe.

To serve:

Let thaw overnight and make pizza per recipe instructions.

Nutritional Information (Per serving):

Calories: 172
Fat: 15 g
Carbohydrate: 1.6 g
Protein: 6 g

SPINACH & SAUSAGE LASAGNA WITH ALMOND FLOUR TORTILLA STRIPS

Makes: 6 servings

All you need:

8 almond flour tortillas cut into strips (See recipe under Bread Category p.80)
1½ cup marinara sauce
½ lb. Italian sausage, mild
2 large bunches of spinach, sautéed in ½ tbsp olive oil
1 cup Provolone cheese, grated
2 cup dry curd cottage cheese
3 tbsp plain yogurt, full fat
¼ tsp salt
1/8 tsp pepper
3 tbsp dried parsley
2 tsp dried basil
2 tbsp parmesan cheese, grated

Alternative:

Substitute 2 cups ricotta cheese in place of dry curd cottage cheese and plain yogurt, if desired.

All you do:

Brown the sausage until cooked through.
Pour in all the sauce except 1/8 cup and bring to a low boil or simmer.
Stir cottage cheese, plain yogurt and seasonings in a separate bowl.
Add the remaining 1/8 cup sauce into the bottom of an 8x11 pan.
Layer the tortilla strips with some overlap.
Spread 1/3 cup of cheese mixture evenly over strips with a spoon.

Add half of the spinach mixture then sprinkle the provolone cheese and finish with 1/3 of the meat sauce.
Continue to follow these layers until ingredients are used up.
Top with parmesan cheese.
Bake for approximately 25 minutes or until cheese is bubbly and lightly golden brown.
Let stand for 10-15 minutes to allow juices to come together.

Freezing Instructions:

Once lasagna is cool, cover the pan with cling wrap then foil.
Label and date the lasagna.
Store in freezer for up to 6 months.

To use:

Let thaw in the refrigerator overnight then heat through.

Nutritional Information (Per serving):

Calories: 276
Fat: 41 g
Carbohydrates: 15 g
Protein: 31 g

SPAGHETTI SQUASH LASAGNA

Makes: 16 servings

All you need:

30 slices whole milk mozzarella cheese
1 large jar (24 oz) marinara sauce
32 oz whole milk ricotta cheese
2 large spaghetti squash, cut in half and de-seeded
3 lbs ground beef, 80/20 or 70/30

All you do:

Preheat oven to 375°F.
Cut the spaghetti squash in half and lay face down in a large baking dish filled with 1-2 inches of water.
Cook the squash for approximately 45 minutes or until soft.
While baking, brown the ground beef until no longer pink.
In a large saucepan, combine meat and sauce and heat through.
Use a fork to scrape out flesh from spaghetti squash until spaghetti consistency.
In a large greased pan, start with a layer of squash, then meat sauce, sliced mozzarella, ricotta and repeat steps.
Bake until lasagna starts to bubble and cheese is lightly golden brown.

Freezing Instructions:

Once lasagna is cooked, remove from oven and let sit at room temperature until cooled down.
Simply wrap with cling wrap then foil.
Label and date the lasagna with cooking instructions.
Place in freezer for up to 3 months.

To serve:

Let thaw overnight in refrigerator then let heat through in the oven before serving.

Nutritional Information (Per serving):

Calories: 438
Fat: 29 g
Carbohydrates: 9 g
Protein: 44g

BREAKFASTS

BACON CHEESE MUFFINS

Makes: 12 servings
Serving size: 1 muffin

All you need:

6 large eggs
6 oz heavy cream
2 cup broccoli florets, chopped
½ cup cheddar cheese, shredded
12 slices bacon
Salt, pepper and garlic powder, to taste
3 slices cheddar cheese

All you do:

Cook bacon until slightly crisp.
Wrap one piece of bacon in each sprayed tin, around the edges.
Pan-fry the broccoli in the bacon grease until crisp-tender.
Add broccoli to the muffin tins.
In a small bowl, whisk cream, eggs and spices.
Pour mixture into each muffin, about ¾ full.
Cook for 20 minutes at 350°F until the top is lightly brown and the muffins are set.

Freezing Instructions:

Allow muffins to cool.
Wrap with cling wrap then foil.

Label and date and store in freezer no longer than 3 months.

To serve:

Remove from freezer and let thaw in refrigerator overnight.
Sprinkle cheddar cheese on top.
Heat muffins in oven until warmed.

Nutritional Information (Per serving):

Calories: 162
Fat: 13 g
Carbohydrates: 2 g
Fiber: 1 g
Protein: 10 g

STEVIA ALMOND YOGURT

Makes: 1 serving

All you need:

4 oz regular, full fat sour cream
4-6 drops of Stevia liquid, varied flavors
Thickener (optional) for serving: 1 tbsp almond flour or milled chia

All you do:

Mix sour cream and Stevia liquid until smooth.

Freezing Instructions:

Cover tightly and freeze up to 6 months.

To serve:

Take out of freezer and let thaw in refrigerator.
To improve smooth texture, gently stir in ½ to 1 tbsp of milled chia or almond flour.

Nutritional information (Per serving):

Calories: 243
Fat: 24 g
Protein: 4 g
Carbohydrates: 4 g

BACON, SPINACH & FETA MUFFINS

Makes: 6 servings

All you need:

6 large eggs
3 slices bacon, cooked, chopped
2 cups raw spinach
1 cup crumbled feta cheese
½ cup cheddar cheese
Salt and pepper, to taste

All you do:

Preheat oven to 350°F.
Heat spinach in a microwave safe bowl on high for 1 minute.
Set aside to cool, retaining liquid if desired (see below).
In a separate bowl, whisk eggs thoroughly until frothy consistency.
Stir in feta cheese and shredded cheddar.
Add cooled spinach and chopped bacon to the bowl. Add liquid from spinach if desired for a moister muffin.
Pour mixture into 6 muffin cups.
Bake for 30-35 minutes, or until muffins are set.

Freezing instructions:

Allow muffins to cool on a wire rack.
Add muffins into a ziploc bag or wrap individually in cling wrap then foil.
Label and date.

To use:

To prepare, take muffin (s) out and let thaw in refrigerator overnight.
Heat through in microwave or oven until warmed through.
For added flavor and fat, spread a layer of butter over muffin (s).
Enjoy!

Nutritional information (Per serving):

Calories: 220
Fat: 16 g
Protein: 12 g
Carbohydrates: 3 g

ALMOND RASPBERRY SCONES

Makes: 9 scones

All you need:

2 eggs, beaten
1 cup almond flour
1/3 cup Stevia
1½ tsp baking powder
1½ tsp vanilla extract
½ cup raspberries, chopped

All you do:

Preheat oven to 375°F.
Combine all ingredients except raspberries in a large bowl.
Fold raspberries in gently.
Drop 2-3 tbsp. of batter onto a baking sheet lined with parchment paper.
Bake for 15 minutes or until lightly browned.
Allow to cool at room temperature.

Freezing Instructions:

Once scones are cooled, simply layer them flat in a freezer ziploc bag with baking paper between the layers.
Label and date freezer bag and store in freezer for up to 3 months.

To serve:

Let thaw at room temperature before serving.
Heat through in oven or microwave, if desired.

Nutritional Information (Per serving):

Calories: 91
Fat: 7 g
Carbohydrates: 4 g
Fiber: 2 g
Protein: 4 g

COCONUT PROTEIN WAFFLES

Makes: 6 servings
Serving size: 2 waffles

All you need:

½ cup coconut flour
1 cup whey protein isolate, not concentrate
½ tsp sea salt
1 tbsp aluminum free baking powder
1 ½ cup coconut milk, unsweetened
4 large eggs
4 tbsp coconut oil, melted

All you do:

Preheat waffle iron to medium-high heat.
Sift together dry ingredients.
In a separate bowl, mix together wet ingredients.
Slowly add dry ingredients to wet ingredients.
Spray waffle iron and once heated, make waffles per liking.

Freezing Instructions:

Layer cooled waffles with parchment paper.
Place into freezer ziploc bag and lay flat in freezer. Store in freezer for up to 3 months

To serve:

Add coconut oil to a griddle over medium-high heat and heat through on both sides.
Serve with your favorite toppings

Nutritional Information (Per serving):

Calories: 322
Fat: 19 g
Carbohydrates: 2.5 g
Protein: 37 g

EASY CARB FREE SYRUP

All you need:

½ cup coconut oil, melted
½ cup Stevia
½ cup almond milk, unsweetened

All you do:

Heat coconut oil over medium-high heat.
Stir in Stevia and almond milk, whisking until smooth.
Let set until cool, for a couple minutes.
Pour into jar of choice and cool at room temperature.
Place in refrigerator for no more than 2 weeks
Note: Do not freeze.

Nutritional Information (Per serving, without syrup):

Calories: 144
Fat: 8 g
Carbohydrates: 4 g
Fiber: 2.1 g
Protein: 12.2 g

CREAM CHEESE PANCAKES

Makes: Four 6-inch pancakes
Serving size: 1 pancake

All you need:

3 medium eggs
2 tbsp psyllium husk powder
½ tsp baking powder
¼ cup cream cheese
Cinnamon or nutmeg, to taste
Pinch of salt
1 tsp vanilla extract
Stevia or sweetener of choice, to taste
Toppings: heavy cream, sugar-free maple syrup (optional)
Coconut oil or butter, for cooking

All you do:

Mix all ingredients together just until moistened.
Heat pan with coconut oil or butter on medium-high heat.
Cook until bubbles lightly pop on both sides.
Flip pancakes and cook until golden brown.

Freezing Instructions:

Allow the pancakes to cool completely, to prevent freezer burn.
Layer pancakes between parchment paper segments.
Put divided pancakes in freezer ziploc bag; label and date the bag.
Place in freezer for up to 1-2 months for highest quality.

To serve:

Remove from freezer and let thaw in refrigerator overnight.
Add to nonstick skillet pan and cook until warm.
Serve with desired toppings.

Nutritional Information (Per serving):

Calories: 344
Fat: 29 g
Carbohydrate: 2.5 g
Protein: 17 g

BREAKFAST SAUSAGE AND CHEESE PINWHEELS

Makes: 10 slices plus 2 end pieces

All you need:

1¼ cup 2% mozzarella cheese, melted (block or regular shredded)
4 tbsp butter, melted
7 tbsp almond flour
1 tsp onion powder
1 large egg
8 oz breakfast pork sausage
½ cup cheddar cheese, shredded

All you do:

Preheat oven to 400°F.
Melt mozzarella cheese in microwave, time varies.
In a small bowl, stir almond flour and onion powder together.
Add melted butter, 1 large egg and flour together until thoroughly mixed.
Use hands and form the dough.
Roll dough into a rectangle on a flat surface on wax paper; set aside.
Now roll out breakfast sausage on a layer of parchment paper into a rectangle. (Note: to prevent cross contamination, use a separate rolling pin).
Place the meat layer on top of the dough and to finish spread mozzarella cheese on top.

Freezing Instructions:

Roll dough like a pinwheel and wrap in parchment paper then foil. Label and date the recipe then place in freezer.

To serve:

Let thaw overnight in refrigerator.
With a sharp paring knife, make 10 even slices, not including end pieces.
In a 400°F, bake for 20 minutes to ensure sausage cooks through.

Nutritional Information (Per serving):

Calories: 269
Fat: 21 g
Carbohydrates: 3 g
Protein: 17 g

BREADS

DECADENT ALMOND MUFFINS

Makes: 3 servings of 2 muffins each

(Perfect for breakfast sandwiches, open-faced sandwiches or as a burger bun)

All you need:

¾ cup almond flour (Bob's Red Mill)
2 large eggs
5 tbsp unsalted butter
1 ½ tsp Stevia, optional
1 ½ tsp baking powder

All you do:

Stir the dry ingredients together.
Gradually whisk the eggs in then pour in the melted butter.
Divide batter into 6 muffin holders.
Bake for 12-17 minutes at 350°F, or until the tops are golden brown.
Cool on a wire rack at room temperature.

Freezing Instructions:

Place all muffins in ziploc freezer bag and remove excess air.
Label and date the bag and place flat into freezer.

To serve:

Remove from freezer and microwave muffin for approximately 15 seconds or put them in the refrigerator to thaw overnight.
Once thawed, microwave for 5 seconds.

Spread with butter or peanut butter for added flavor and/or additional fat, if desired.

Nutritional Information (Per 2 muffins):

Calories: 373
Fat: 35 g
Carbohydrate: 7 g
Fiber: 3 g
Protein: 10 g

FOUR INGREDIENT BREAD LOAF

Makes: 10 servings
Serving size: 1 slice

All you need:

3 large eggs
2/3 cup ground almond flour
1½ tsp baking powder
2 tbsp butter, melted

All you do:

Add ingredients to a bowl and whisk just until moistened.
Pour into a greased bread pan.
Pick up bread pan and lightly drop onto counter to evenly disperse bread mix.
Bake in oven for 20 minutes at 375°F.
Let bread cool, and then remove from pan onto cutting board or wire rack.

Freezing Instructions:

Once cooled, wrap in cling wrap and foil. Label and date bread and place in freezer.

To use:

Remove bread from freezer and let thaw at room temperature or in refrigerator, as desired.
Serve with a spread of butter or drizzle of sugar-free maple syrup.
Enjoy with an 8 oz. glass of unsweetened almond milk.

Nutritional Information:

Calories: 283
Fat: 25 g
Carbohydrates: 6 g
Protein: 2 g

ALMOND FLOUR TORTILLAS

Makes: 8 tortillas
Serving size: 1 tortilla

All you need:

2 cup almond flour
2 large eggs
1 tsp olive oil
½ tsp salt

All you do:

Preheat oven to 350°F.
In a bowl, combine all ingredients and knead for 1-2 minutes.
Sprinkle a little almond flour on a flat surface and roll out the dough to about 1/8" inch thick.
Bake for 8 minutes or until golden brown.

Freezing Instructions:

Let tortillas cool.
Layer in between each tortilla a piece of parchment paper cut into a square.
Continue layers of parchment paper and tortillas and place into a ziploc freezer bag.
Label and date the freezer bag then store in freezer for 1-2 months.

To use:

Take out of freezer and let thaw at room temperature before serving.

Nutritional Information (Per serving):

Calories: 39
Fat: 15.8 g
Carbohydrates: 6.1 g
Protein: 7.5 g

ZUCCHINI BREAD

Makes: 10 slices

All you need:

1¾ cup almond flour
1 cup Stevia
2 tsp baking powder
1 tsp ground cinnamon
½ tsp nutmeg
½ tsp salt
¼ tsp ground cloves
1/3 cup coconut oil
2 large eggs
2 tsp pure vanilla
1 cup grated zucchini
½ cup slivered almonds, toasted (optional)

All you do:

Pre-heat oven to 350°F.
Grease and sprinkle almond flour in the bread loaf pan.
Combine all the dry ingredients in one bowl.
Combine all the wet ingredients, including the zucchini and toasted pecans.
Slowly mix the dry ingredients into the wet ingredients. Do not over mix.
Pour batter into prepared bread pan and bake for approximately 40 minutes, or until toothpick comes out clean.
Remove from the oven and cool on countertop.

Freezing Instructions:

Wrap in cling wrap then foil.
Label and date then place in freezer.

To use:

Thaw in refrigerator then microwave for 5 seconds.
Or take out of freezer and microwave for 15-20 seconds.

Nutritional Information (Per serving):

Calories: 214
Fat: 27.75 g
Protein: 9.2 g
Carbohydrates 10 g

DESSERTS & SNACKS

CHOCOLATE COCONUT SQUARES

Makes: 12 bars
Serving size: 1 bar

All you need:

Bottom Coconut Layer:

2 cups shredded coconut, unsweetened
1/3 cup coconut oil, unrefined and melted
2 droppers liquid Stevia

Chocolate topping layer:

3 squares baker's chocolate, unsweetened
1 tbsp coconut oil
2 droppers liquid Stevia

All you do:

Bottom layer:

Place all bottom coconut layer ingredients into a food processor.
Pulse until the dough forms and pulls away from sides.
Scrape dough from the sides as needed.
Press the coconut dough mixture into a 9x5 loaf pan (silicon) and set in freezer.

Top layer:

Heat coconut oil and baker's chocolate in microwave-safe bowl just until melted.

Stir in Stevia drops.
Take bottom coconut layer out of freezer and pour chocolate layer on top.
Place pan back into the freezer until solid, approximately 30 minutes.
Take out of the freezer and turn pan over to empty the dessert.
Cut bars into 12 squares.

Freezing Instructions:

Can be stored in a large ziploc bag in freezer.

Serving Suggestion:

Add in slivered almonds for a crunchy bar and for increased fat and protein.

Nutritional information (Per serving):

Calories: 216
Fat: 22 g
Carbohydrates: 2 g
Protein: 2 g

ALMOND CHEESECAKE

Makes: 16 servings

All you need:

Crust:

1 cup almond flour
2 tbsp butter, melted

Filling:

3 bricks cream cheese (1½ lbs.)
¼ cup Stevia Liquid
1 tsp vanilla extract
¼ tsp salt
4 eggs
¼ cup lemon juice
1 tbsp zest of lemon
¼ cup heavy whipping cream

Topping:

1 cup sour cream
2 tbsp lemon juice, freshly squeezed
1 tbsp lemon zest
1 tbsp Stevia liquid dropper

All you do:

Crust:

Simply mix both ingredients together and press into a spring-form pan.
Bake for 6-8 minutes at 375°F until lightly golden brown.
Remove from oven and set aside.

Filling:

Beat cream cheese until whipped.
Add in remaining ingredients and mix well.
Pour mixture over cooled crust.
Place the pan into a larger pan that is filled with 1-2 inches of water, for even baking.
Bake for 50-60 minutes at 350°F, or until cheesecake is firm.

Topping (make during baking):

Stir all four ingredients together in a small bowl.
After cheesecake is done, spread topping over cake and bake for an additional 10 minutes.
Cool cheesecake for 2 hours or more.
Refrigerate overnight.

Freezing Instructions:

Wrap cheesecake with cling wrap then foil.
Label and date the cheesecake and place in freezer.

To serve:

Remove from freezer and let thaw overnight in refrigerator before serving.

Optional:

Add a dollop of whipped topping, which will add 100 calories, 11 g fat and 1 g carb.

Nutritional information (Per serving):

Calories: 260
Fat: 23 g
Carbohydrates: 4 g
Protein: 5 g

ALMOND BUTTER COCONUT FUDGE BARS

Makes: 10 bars
Serving size: 1 bar

All you need:

½ cup coconut oil, unrefined
1 cup almond butter, unsalted
3 tbsp Stevia + 1 tsp almond or vanilla extract
½ tsp salt
½ cup shredded coconut, unsweetened

All you do:

Line an 8x8-baking pan with parchment paper.
Using a double broiler or microwave, melt coconut oil, Stevia/extract, salt and almond butter just until melted or smooth.
Remove from heat and gently fold in coconut.
Pour mixture into the baking pan.
Let set in freezer for up to 2 hours or until firm.
Once hardened, remove from freezer and lift parchment paper to lift bars out.
Cut into square bars.

Freezing Instructions:

Keep bars separate with parchment paper.
Store in freezer in a sealed container.

Nutritional Information (Per serving):

Calories: 192
Fat: 20 g
Carbohydrates: 2 g
Protein: 3 g

QUEST BAR COOKIES

Makes: 1 serving
Serving size: 8 small balls

All you need:

Quest Protein Bar, preferably Chocolate Chip Cookie Dough

All you do:

Preheat oven to 450°F.
Heat Quest bar in microwave for approximately 10 seconds.
Divide bar into 8 equal parts.
Roll into balls and bake on a cookie sheet for a couple minutes.

Freezing Instructions:

Note: Buy a large box of Quest Bars to store extra in the freezer. Simply add cooled balls to a freezer ziploc bag and lay flat in freezer.

Nutritional information (Per serving):

Calories: 190
Fat: 8 g
Carbohydrates: 12.5g
Protein: 21 g
Fiber: 17g

AVOCADO PRESERVES

Makes: 25 servings (1/5 medium avocado)

All you need:

5 ripe avocados
5 tbsp lemon juice

All you do:

Slice the avocados in half and discard pits.
Scoop the fresh from the peels with a spoon.
Place pitted and peeled avocados in a bowl.
Mash well with one tbsp. of lemon juice for each avocado.

Freezing Instructions:

Spoon mixture into a gallon sized zip top bag, squeezing out all the air before sealing.
Label and date the bag.
May be safely store in freezer up to one year.
Complements well with tacos, pork, chicken, smoothies and even chocolate pudding!

Nutritional Information (Per serving):

Calories: 50
Fat: 4.5 g
Carbohydrates: 3 g
Protein: 0 g

ALSO BY SKYE HOWARD FOR THE KETOGENIC DIET:

KETO SMOOTHIES & SHAKES -

40 RECIPES - HI FAT / LOW CARB / VARIED PROTEIN TO MEET ALL PROTEIN INTAKE REQUIREMENTS

KETO ONE POT MEALS

45 EASY KETO RECIPES FOR SKILLET, CROCKPOT AND OVEN

OTHER TITLES BY SCG PUBLISHING

The Migraine Diet Cookbook by Michelle Strong

Migraine Safe Smoothies by Michelle Strong

Chilli Jam Recipes by Amanda Kent

HIIT: High Intensity Interval Training by Steve Ryan (BSCExercise&NutritionBScSport)

Made in the USA
San Bernardino, CA
17 January 2018